MAR 2 0 2007

.I

D1549138

2006

I Just Am

I Just Am

A STORY OF DOWN SYNDROME AWARENESS AND TOLERANCE

by Bryan and Tom Lambke

with a foreword by
Shannon D. R. Ringenbach, Ph.D.
Department of Kinesiology Arizona State University

and introduction by
Cheryl Rogers-Barnett
daughter of Roy Rogers and Dale Evans

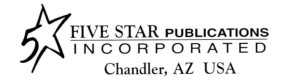
FIVE STAR PUBLICATIONS
INCORPORATED
Chandler, AZ USA

Linda F. Radke, President
FIVE STAR PUBLICATIONS, INC.
P.O. Box 6698
Chandler, Arizona 85246-6698
480-940-8182
www.FiveStarPublications.com
www.IJustAm.org

Library of Congress Cataloging-in-Publication Data

Lambke, Bryan, 1981-
 I just am / by Bryan and Tom Lambke ; with a foreword by Shannon D.R. Ringenbach and introduction by Cheryl Rogers-Barnett.
    p. cm.
 ISBN 978-1-58985-020-0
 1. Lambke, Bryan, 1981- 2. Down syndrome–Patients–United States–Biography. I. Lambke, Tom, 1955- II. Title.
 RJ506.D68L36 2006
 362.196'8588420092–dc22

2005030333

ISBN: 978-1-58985-020-0
Manufactured in Canada
10 9 8 7 6 5 4 3 2 1

Cover and interior design: Janet Bergin
Photography: Sarah Elsasser, Karen and Tom Lambke
Photos used in the introduction courtesy of the Cheryl Rogers-Barnett collection.

CONTENTS

JUST WHEN YOU THINK YOU HAVE LEARNED
WHAT YOU NEED TO KNOW IN LIFE,
SOMEONE SPECIAL COMES INTO IT AND
SHOWS JUST HOW MUCH MORE THERE IS.

— author unknown

SPONSORS

DOWN SYNDROME NETWORK ARIZONA

DR. SHANNON RINGENBACH

MARY JO and KEN LAMBKE

CHARLOTTE DAVIDGE (TOM'S MOM)

This book is written in memory of Bryan's grandfathers,

Joe Capezio and Tom Lambke, who both passed away in 2001.

Grandpa Capezio never met a person he did not like, and Grandpa

Lambke instilled in me the courage to try everything. You both showed

an awareness of Bryan's disability and helped guide others in helping us

to raise him. You should be proud of his accomplishments.

We miss you both and think of you often. May you rest in peace.

DEDICATION

This book is dedicated to the two ladies in our lives who we love with as much love as our hearts can hold. Bryan's sister Shauna, who still only sees the good in people, a quality we hope she retains forever, please do not change. Bryan's Mom and my beautiful wife, Karen, who has supported my decisions to journey in whatever direction I have chosen and has always been there for both of us.

It is dedicated to our families, especially Bryan's grandparents. When Bryan was born, Karen's parents, Josephine and Joe, and my parents, Charlotte and Tom, all displayed a remarkable tolerance and acceptance of Bryan and his disability. They taught us the courage and humility it took to raise Bryan in a world full of prejudice and ignorance. Their message of love is deeply appreciated.

This book is also dedicated to all of those individuals with Down syndrome who have the same feelings, who share the same dreams, and who deserve to have the same happiness as I have been blessed.

This book is written for those who think of Down syndrome as a disease, who believe one can die from Down syndrome, and especially for those who still refer to someone with Down syndrome as a Mongoloid. If this book can change those misconceptions, we will be ecstatic.

PLANT A SEED AND WATCH IT GROW.

INSPIRE GREATNESS IN OTHERS

AND FULFILL A NEED.

IF YOU SHED A TEAR,

HUG YOURSELF,

BECAUSE YOU ARE A COMPASSIONATE PERSON.

ACKNOWLEDGEMENTS

Thanks to our good friend, Linda Radke, President of Five Star Publications, and her staff, for their enormous assistance and commitment to excellence. It has been a joy working with you and getting to know you and your wonderful family.

Thank you to Down Syndrome Network Arizona and their President, Janet Romo, whose leadership and people skills are unequaled. Your excitement and motivation have been an inspiration to us and we value your friendship. Thanks also to Dr. Shannon Ringenbach and her research in Down syndrome which has established her permanently in her field. We have enjoyed working with you and getting to know your family and wish you luck in your future endeavors.

A special thanks to all of our good friends, most of whom are featured in some of the pictures including: Mike and Dean Alber, Scott Althoff, Kevin Griffin, Rob Harris, Nicki Hawk, Chad Herd, Gena Horne, Steve (Bulldog) Hunter, Jessica (J.J.) Jacobus, Scott Kleck, Judy Lins, Keith Mallett, Jamie Mote, Michael Tom, Jennifer Twitchell, Danny Vukobratovich, Larry West, Nicole Wilkes and Michael Williams.

A very special thanks also to all the administrators, teachers and instructional assistants at Corona del Sol High School who not only helped to make Bryan's high school years a happy and productive experience, but who have also helped to make me a better person and teacher to students with disabilities. This includes Donna Baker, Kirsten Barnett, Barb Carter, Pat Cahalan, Shannon Corcoron, Jim Denton, Tammy Forrest, Ed Garcia, Mitch Gonzalez, Hope Grunow, Kim Gumbert, Beth Heerding, David Himmelstein, Rosanne Hopwood, Cathy Lolly, Sean McDonald, Linda Nelson, Dan Nero, Maria Renteria, Dianne Saints, Dan Salas, Lindsey Scarborough, Katie Sheffield, Steve Shively, Jayelee Stone, Amy Taylor, Dave Vibber, Patty Vogel, Missy West, Steve Wilbur and Marilyn Williams.

An extra special thanks to our good friend, Sarah Elsasser, who was our photographer in this project. She is a very special young lady with a heart of gold who will achieve much in her lifetime.

To all who have someone in their lives with Down syndrome and to those individuals with Down syndrome, your patience and will is inspiring.

ABOUT THE AUTHORS

Bryan is now twenty-three years old and holds two jobs. Monday through Friday, he is employed in the work center at TCH, the Center for Habilitation, where he sorts x-rays for shredding and helps run the conveyor belt. On Friday evenings and Sunday afternoons, he works as a meeter/greeter at the Chandler AMF Bowling Center. He meets and greets customers at the door where he passes out flyers, helps clean tables and puts away bowling balls. His dreams are to get a license and drive, live on his own, and get married. Bryan has achieved so much already that these goals certainly do not seem impossible. He continues to participate and compete in Special Olympics, particularly bowling, swimming and basketball. Bryan also goes out on dates and has special girlfriends named Nicki and Nicole.

Tom is also the author of *Spirit, Courage and Resolve…a Special Olympics Athlete's Road to Gold*, a story about Bryan's achievements and successes. He is now an Instructional Assistant in Special Education at Corona del Sol High School in Bryan's old class and still umpires baseball and softball regularly. His goal is to go back to school for his teacher's certificate and teach Special Ed. Tom has finally realized his place in life working with people with disabilities and is extremely proud to do so. He is also lucky to have an incredible spouse of twenty-eight years, Karen, who understands his desires and has allowed him to do what he needs to do in life. They are also the proud parents of twenty-year old Shauna, who works with individuals with special needs at an elementary school and is taking college courses toward a degree in nursing.

IN THE MORNING ASK YOURSELF,

"WHAT GOOD SHALL I DO TODAY?"

AS THE DAY DRAWS TO A CLOSE ASK YOURSELF,

"WHAT GOOD HAVE I DONE TODAY?"

— Ben Franklin

FOREWORD

By Shannon D. R. Ringenbach, Ph.D.

I smile whenever I think of Bryan and Tom Lambke; probably because they are always smiling, always available to help, and always caring. I am an Associate Professor at Arizona State University in the Department of Kinesiology studying the most effective method of providing instructions to persons with DS to perform different types of movements. My hope is that adults with Down syndrome will continue to learn in a manner that is easiest for them and the least frustrating for caregivers. While I am a scientist, I have noticed that parents of people with Down syndrome often know things that it takes scientists years to learn, and the Lambke's are a perfect example of this. They have fostered learning many things in many ways in Bryan, and Bryan has flourished. It is clear that Bryan has learned a lot, but he has probably taught many people more. The present book is one more example of this. Bryan has taught me to listen (I have never known him to interrupt someone speaking) and he has taught me to work hard (he has more jobs and commitments than most people). I have no doubt that in this book Bryan will teach you something. This book questions what normal really is. After being around Bryan, I don't think he is normal; he is better than normal.

PREFACE

By Tom Lambke

As Linda Radke, her staff at Five Star Publications, and I were putting the finishing touches on this book before bringing it to press, I visited our local library and checked out a copy of *Angel Unaware*, written by Dale Evans, Cheryl Rogers-Barnett's mother. For those of you too young to know, Dale Evans was married to Roy Rogers, one of the most famous cowboys of the 20th Century, and they were one of the most famous and loved couples of their generation. *Angel Unaware* was written as if their daughter Robin Elizabeth was speaking from heaven about her short experience on earth. She explains how God had sent her "down there" to teach her mom and dad patience and understanding about her disability, and to teach others. I could not put the book down until I read it all.

I wish someone had given me this book when Bryan was born. Although it was written in 1953 and Dale Evans refers to her daughter as Mongoloid (an accepted term back then), *Angel Unaware* invoked feelings in me I had not felt in a long time. I do not consider myself to be a devoutly religious man, but this powerful little book made me realize that my wife and I have been guided all along since our son Bryan was born. Whenever people said we had been chosen to be Bryan's parents for a reason, I always felt compelled to brush them off with statements like, "We are not more special than anyone else." I really believed that, too.

Now I truly understand that Bryan was sent to us as a messenger—to teach us how to change attitudes and perceptions about people with any disability, not just Down syndrome. While reading *Angel Unaware*, I felt as if Robin Elizabeth were speaking to me. I finally realized why I am, and who I am, and that I will continue to spread the word.

One fact that really hit home was discovering that Robin Elizabeth Rogers was born August 26, 1950. Our good friend Chris Burke, the actor from the television show *Life Goes On*, was born August 26, 1965. I was born August 26, 1955. I do not believe in coincidences.

I do believe all doctors and parents of babies with a disability should be given a copy of *Angel Unaware*. Your child will change your life—this book will help.

INTRODUCTION

When my baby sister Robin Elizabeth was diagnosed with Down syndrome, our parents were advised to find a hospital where she could live out the short life expectancy associated with her condition. "Don't take her home...she will never recognize you...she will never live past her 20th birthday...don't get attached...getting attached will just break your heart." That was the prevailing feeling and advice of the medical profession towards children with Down's in 1950.

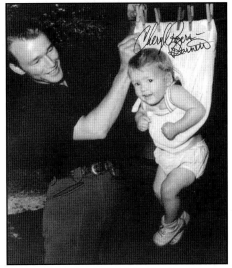

Cheryl and her dad, Roy Rogers

Our parents, Roy Rogers and Dale Evans, refused to take their advice. They insisted upon bringing Robin into our home, where she had two sisters (Cheryl, 10 and Linda Lou, 7) and two brothers (Tom, 23 and Dusty, 4). For the next two years, Robin had as normal a life as a baby with health problems could have while living in a family with world-famous parents. She was never hidden from the spotlight but was protected as much as possible from too many people and too much excitement at one time.

Even though Robin didn't live to see her second birthday, for the fifty years following her death, her short life has exerted a positive influence upon untold thousands of people. When Mom wrote her first book and told Robin's story in *Angel Unaware,* no one could predict that 50 years later, Mom's little book would still be the book that friends and relatives would give when a handicapped child was born or a beloved child was lost.

All proceeds from "Angel" have been used to fund research on Down syndrome, as Mom always said that *Angel Unaware* was a gift from God. she never could have written it herself. I hope you will find Bryan's story to be a gift to you and those you love. That it will enrich your lives and give you a better understanding and appreciation of how truly special these "special children" are.

Cheryl Rogers-Barnett

Q&A With Tom Lambke and Cheryl Rogers-Barnett

Tom: How old were you when Robin Elizabeth was born?
Cheryl: Ten
Tom: Did you know that she was different right away?
Cheryl: We were told that our new baby sister had health problems, that the doctors had advised them not to bring her home, but they were going to bring her home anyway. That we would have to be very quiet around her and not do anything to startle her because she had a

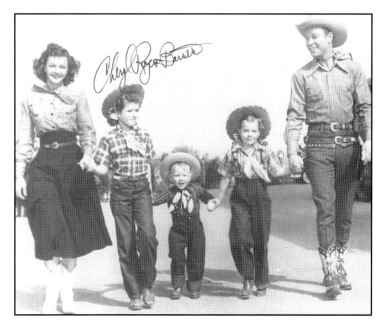

Dale, Cheryl, Dusty, Linda Lou and Roy.

very weak heart.

Tom: How did your other siblings react to her?

Cheryl: Linda Lou and I loved her. I was ten and Linda Lou was seven so we wanted to play with her but knew she was too weak. Dusty was only four and a boy, so I don't know how much he could understand, except that he had to be quiet when she was around.

Tom: Did your friends know about your "different" sister?

Cheryl: Yes. But we never played in an area that Robin would be disturbed.

Tom: How were your parents informed of her disability?

Cheryl: I don't know how they told Dad. He knew about Robin's problems first. They didn't tell Mom for a couple of days but since they weren't bringing the baby to her, she knew that something was up but when she did see Robin she thought she looked like Dad as he had very squinty eyes. They finally told her that Robin had Down syndrome, a weak heart and other problems that sometimes go with the syndrome.

Tom: Were they told to institutionalize her or give her away?

Cheryl: They were told to institutionalize her and to not let themselves get attached to her as she could never lead a normal life, would probably never recognize them and would probably not live past 20.

Tom: What kind of health problems did she have, and were they a factor in her dying so young?

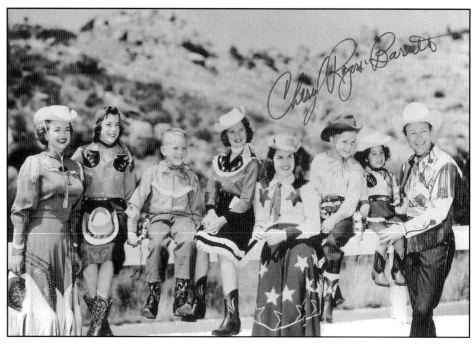

The Rogers Family

Cheryl: Robin had a bad heart valve making her heart very weak but, at that time, open-heart surgery was not performed on children younger than five. The hole at the top of her palate did not close and she had a weakened immune system. She also had weak hip joints (something her brother, Tom's oldest daughter also had). She wore a bar with shoes at the ends to help with her hips. Even though she had a full-time nurse with her, no one recognized that she had gotten polio until she stopped making progress crawling. She was diagnosed and seemed to be doing fine when the rest of us came down with mumps. Robin caught the mumps and then it went into brain-fever.

Tom: Because of their celebrity status, did people react to Robin in a more positive attitude than they would have if she was not the daughter of a famous couple?

Cheryl: I don't know. The only people who saw Robin were family and very close friends. Strangers seemed to upset her.

Tom: How did your parents treat her?

Cheryl: Like the sweet, loving little girl she was.

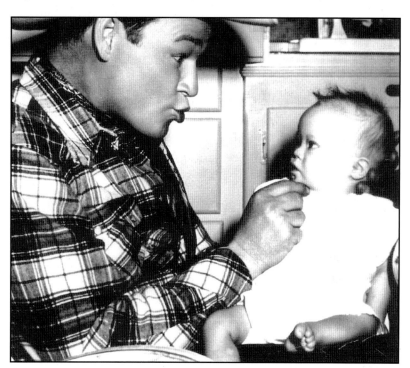

Roy Rogers and Robin Elizabeth

Tom: Was she hidden from others or brought out in the open?

Cheryl: She was not hidden from others but they also didn't put her in situations where she wasn't comfortable. She was included in family pictures that were made available to the fan magazines of that time. But because of her immune system and heart problems, she was not taken out in public.

Tom: Are there any other relatives in the immediate family with disabilities, Down syndrome or otherwise?

Cheryl: Yes, one of the great-grandchildren has Rhett's syndrome and another has been diagnosed as autistic. Diabetes is also prevalent in my brother, Tom's family.

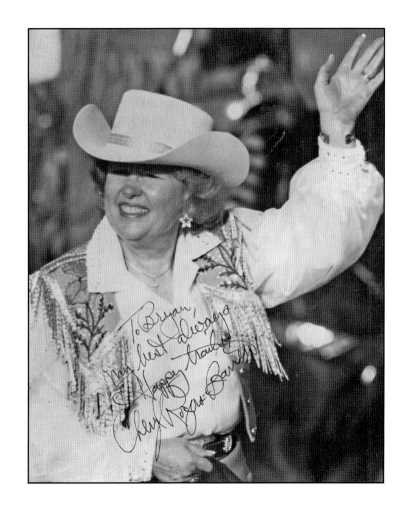

To Bryan,
my best always,
Happy trails,
Dale Rogers Barnett

This is a story about a young man with

Down syndrome.

These are his thoughts and feelings

regarding his disability.

It is written with help from his dad and

much love.

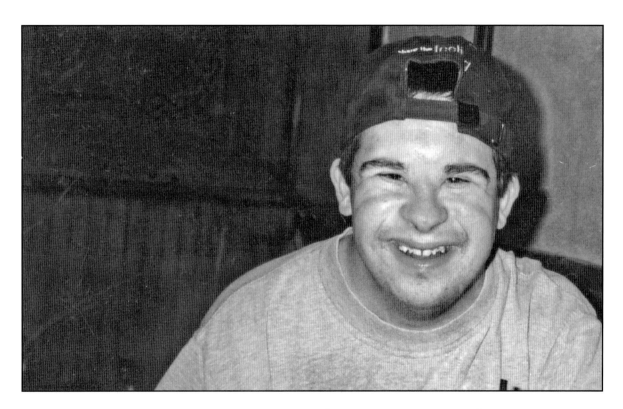

My name is Bryan. I have a disability.

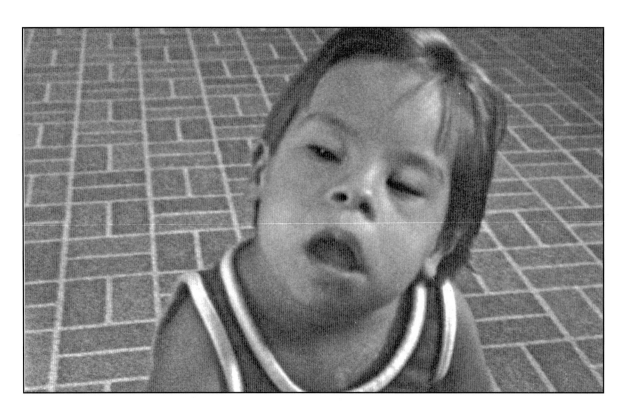

It is not my fault. I just am.

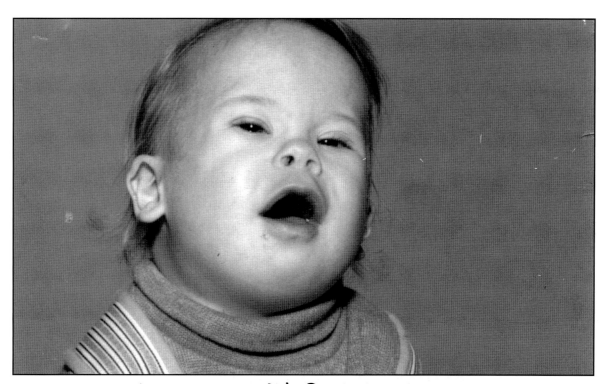

I was born with Down syndrome.
There are a lot of people with it.

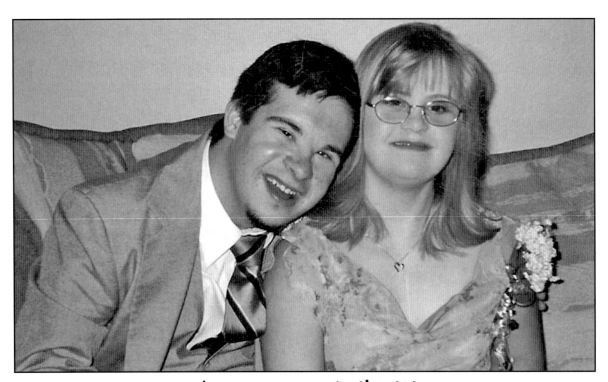

We have many similarities.
But we are also all very unique.

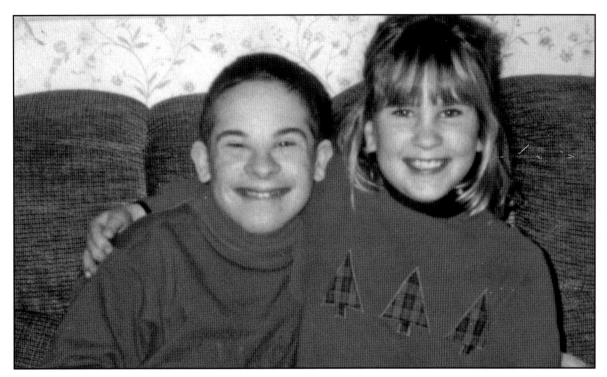

Down syndrome is having an extra chromosome.
It makes me look different than others.

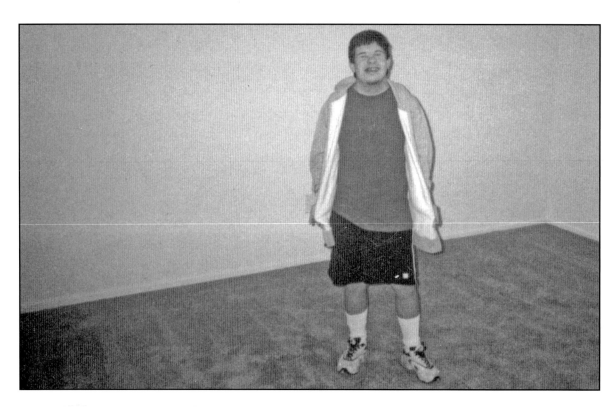

I don't feel different. I just am.

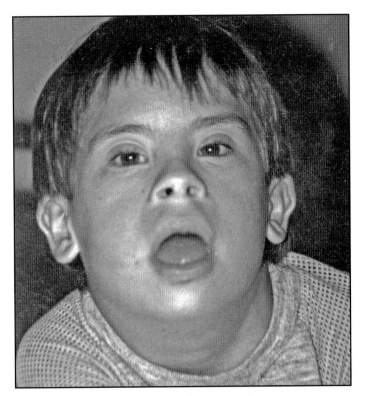

I am not stupid.
But I am slow.

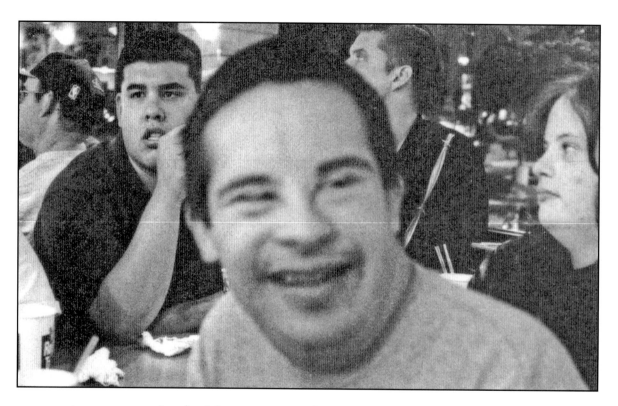

I do not look like normal. But what is normal?

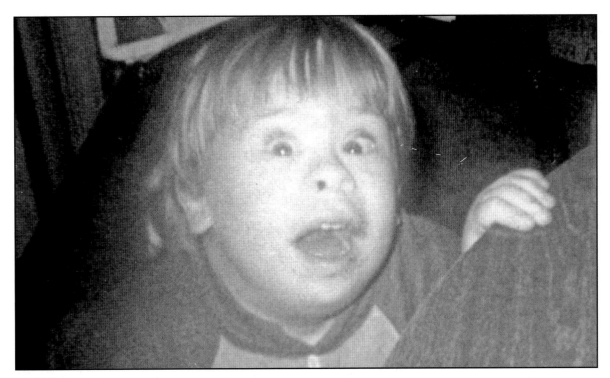

Down syndrome is not a disease.
And it is not contagious.

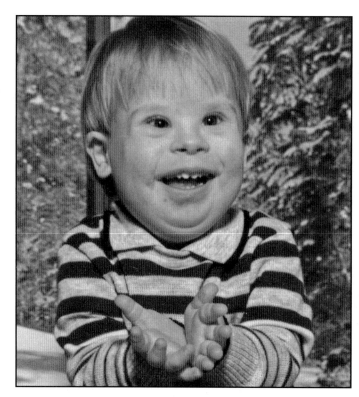

It is not hereditary.
It is not normal.

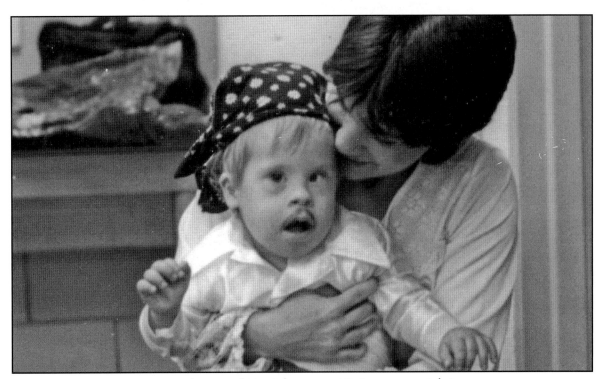

My parents thought they did something wrong.
But they didn't.

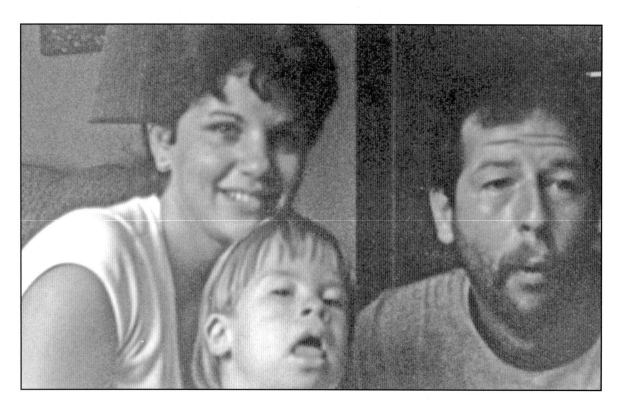

So they raised me like normal. But what is normal?

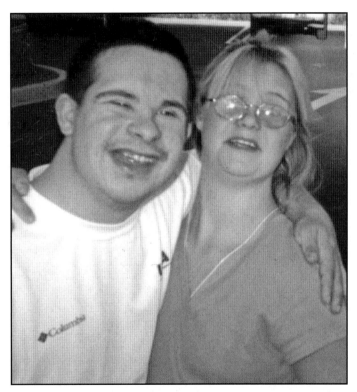

Normal is feeling happy.
I am happy.

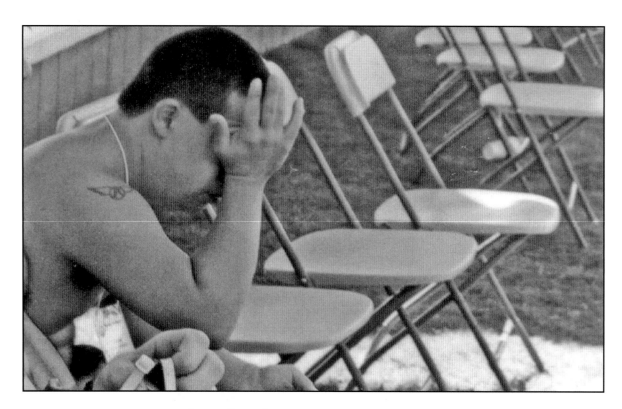

Normal is feeling sad. I can be sad.

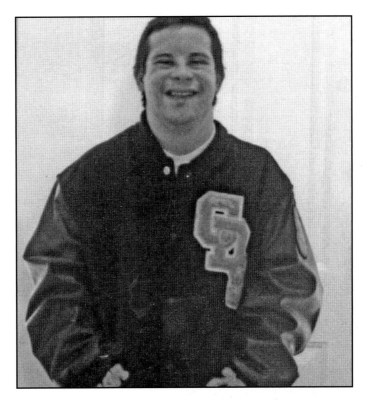

Normal means going to school. I gradu-
ated from Corona del Sol High School.

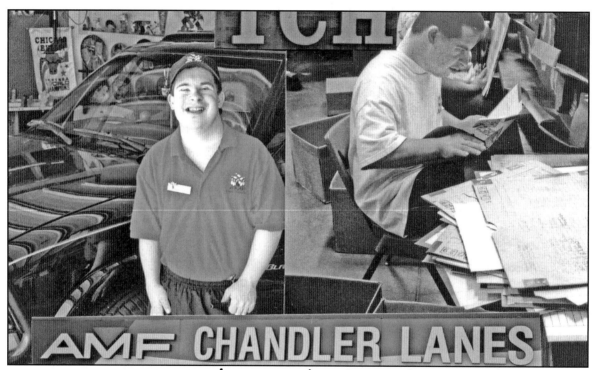

Normal means having a job.
I have two jobs and go to work every day.

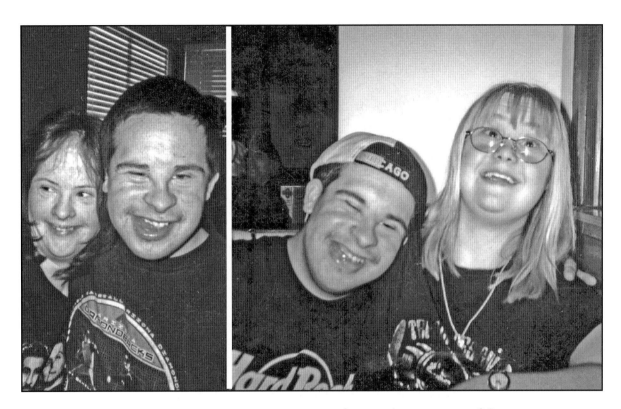

I am twenty-three years old. I have girlfriends.

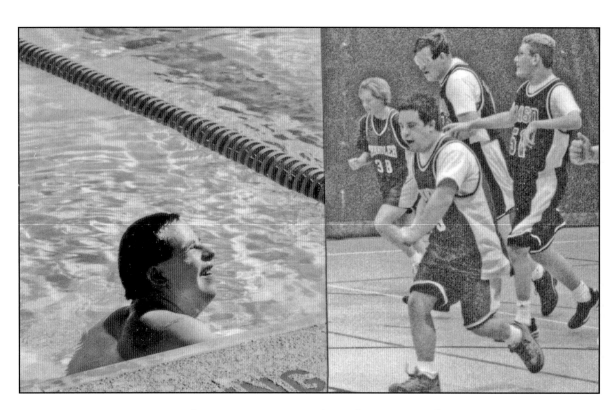

I play sports. I feel normal.

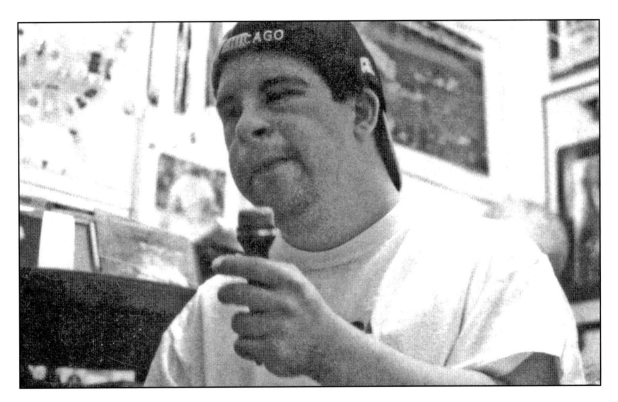

I like watching television. I love listening to rock and roll.

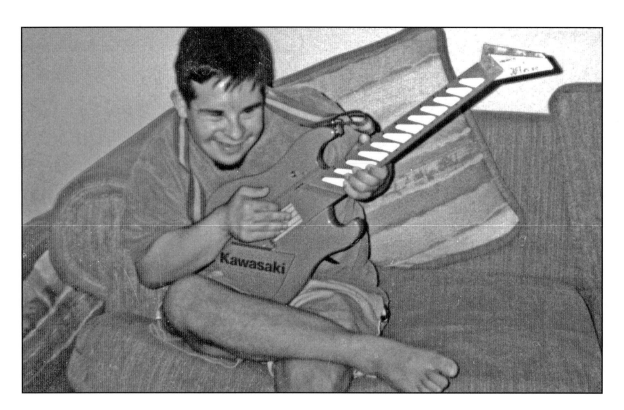

I want to be normal. What is normal?

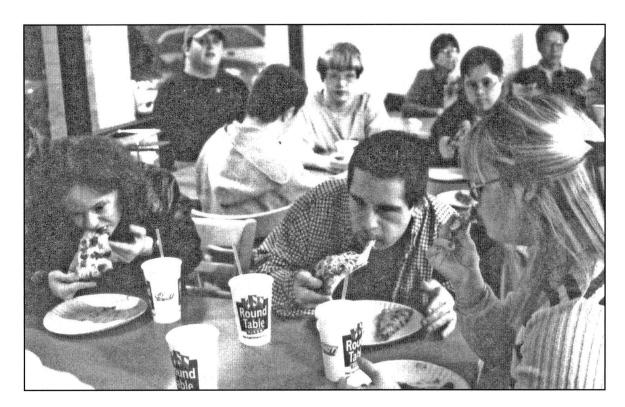

I like nachos. I love pizza.

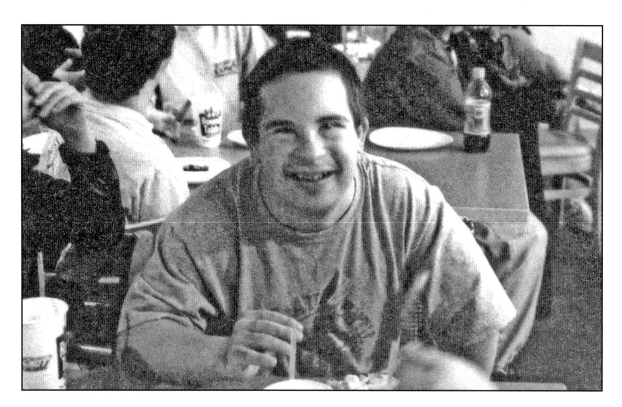

I don't like veggies. Seems normal.

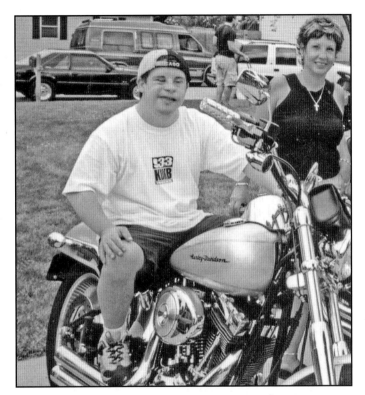

I want a motorcycle.

I want a car.

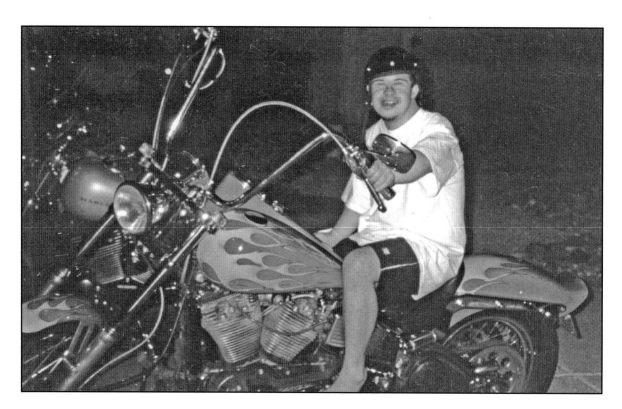

I want a license. I want to be normal.

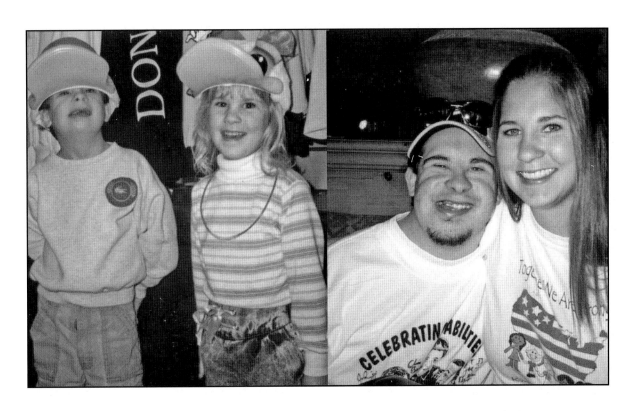

I have a sister I love dearly. I have a life.

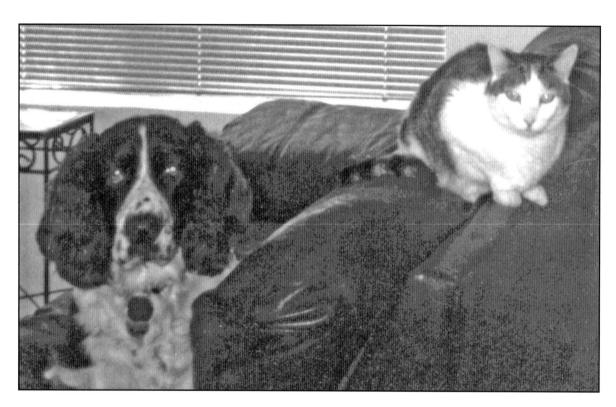

I have a dog and cat I love, too. I am normal.

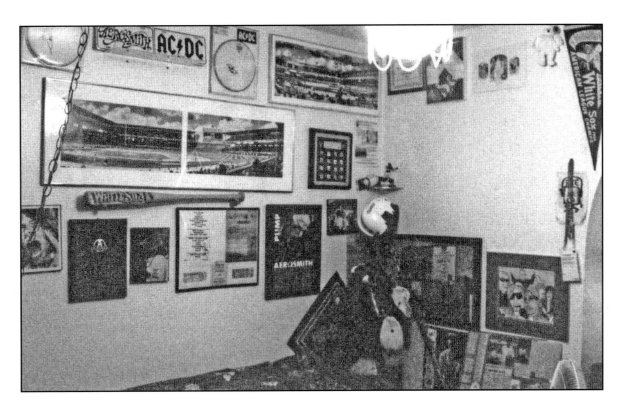

I have my own bedroom. Sometimes it is a mess.

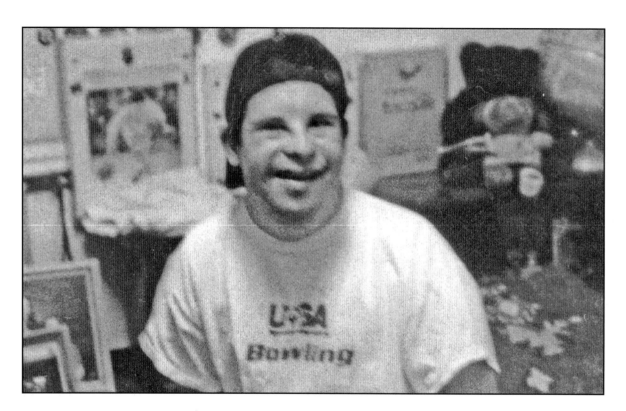

I try to keep it clean. That is normal.

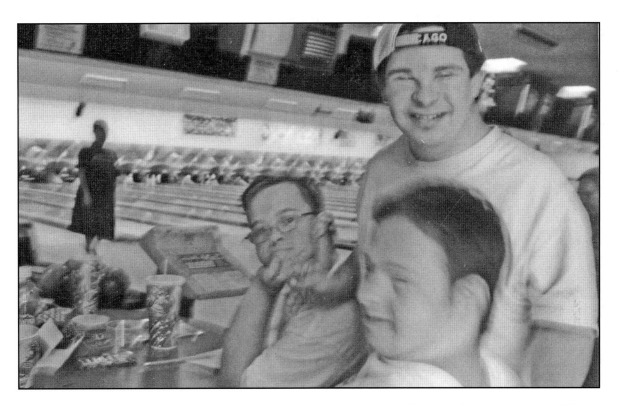

Others call me handicapped. Why label me at all?

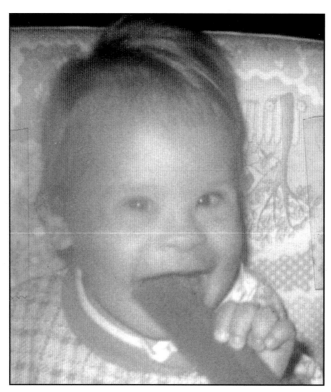

I don't call you names.
Why can't I be normal?

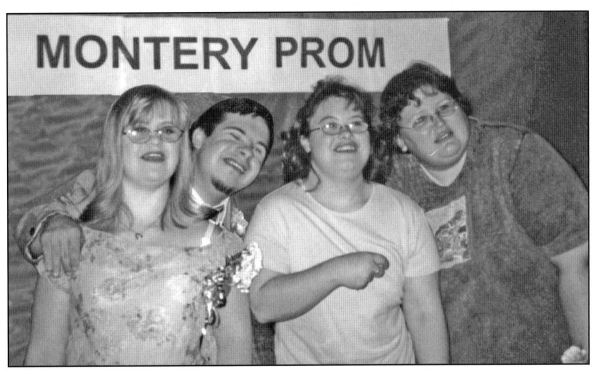

People with Down syndrome can do anything you can do. We have the same chances you have.

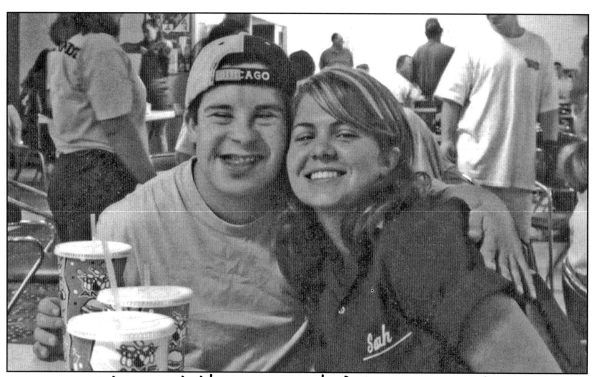

We want the same choices you want.

To us, we are just like you.

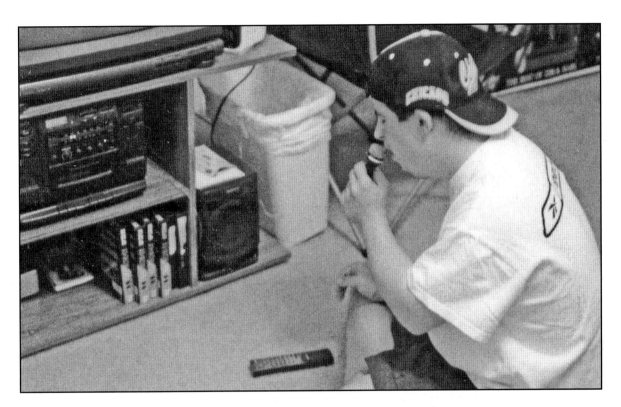

I like to sing. Maybe not in key.

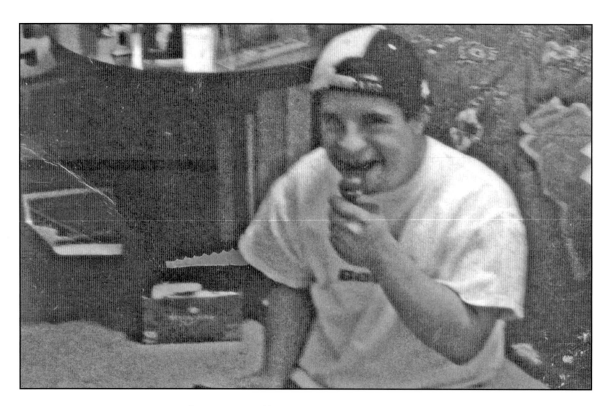

But I know all the words. Do you?

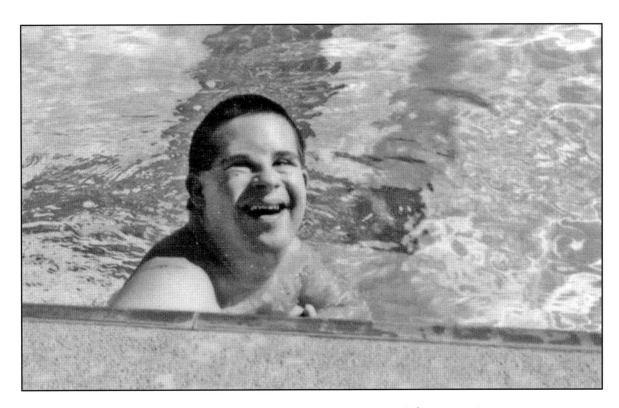

I like the water. I can swim like a fish.

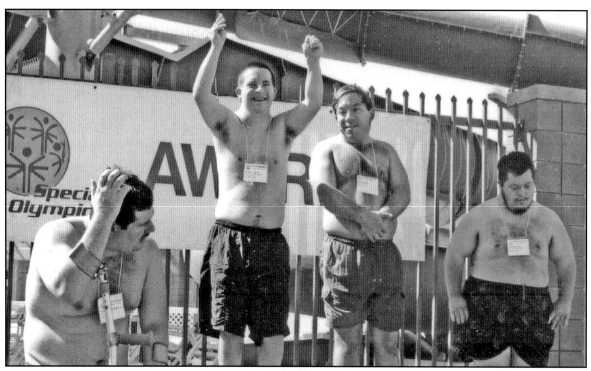

I can hold my breath underwater for a long time.
How long can you?

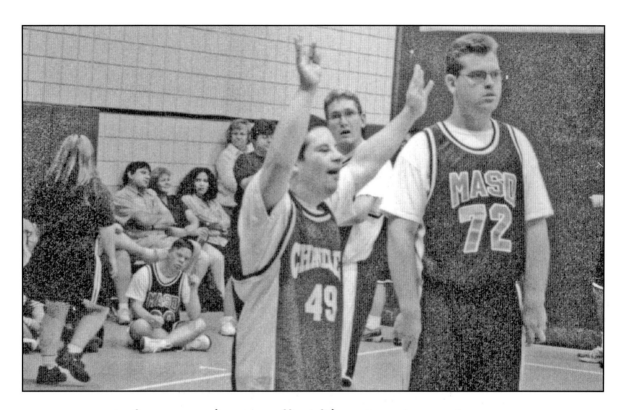

I play basketball. I like to shoot hoops.

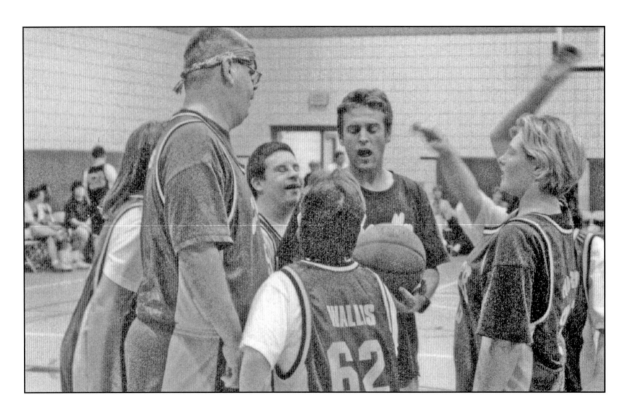

I don't make all my shots. Do you?

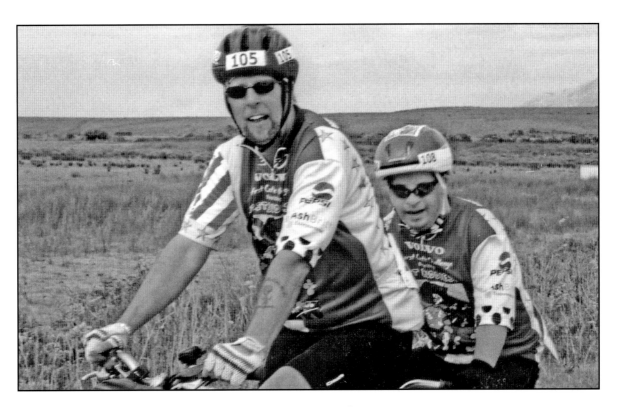

I can ride a bike. I like to go fast.

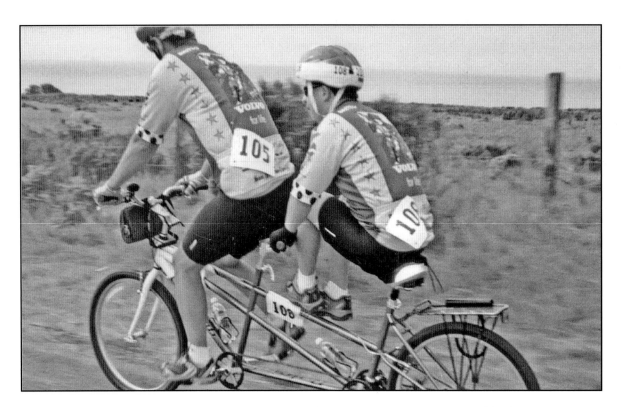

Stopping can be a problem. But it is still fun.

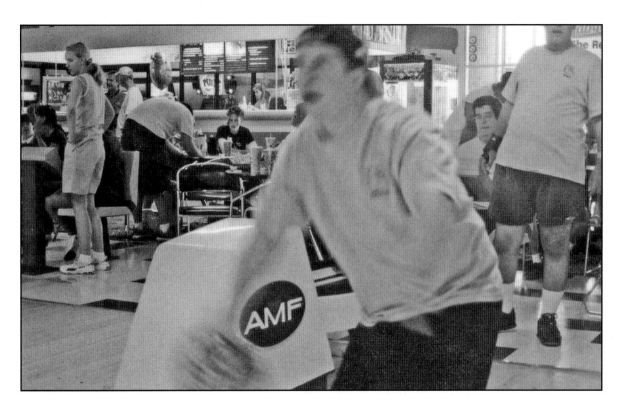

I love to bowl. Sometimes in the hundreds.

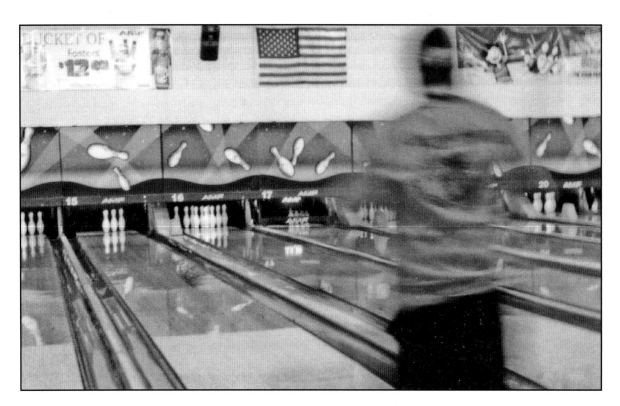

I am not perfect. Are you?

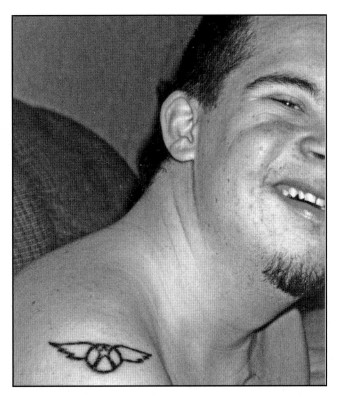

I have a tattoo.
It hurt a little.

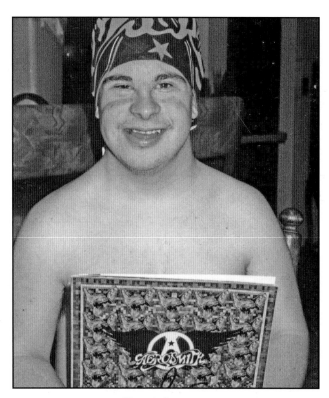

But I really like Aerosmith.
Do you have any tats?

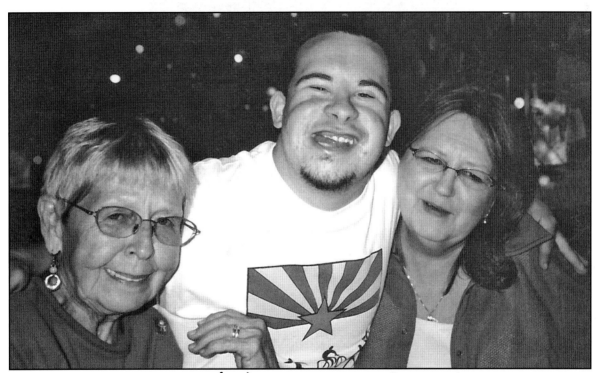

I recently had my ear pierced.
Courtesy of my Aunt Linda and Grandma.

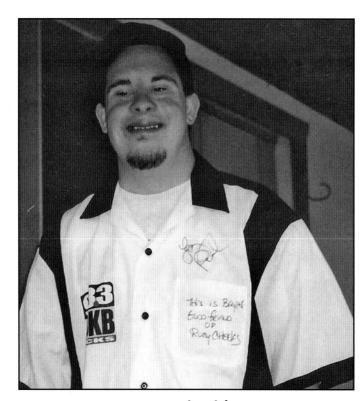

Most people like it.
I think it looks rad.

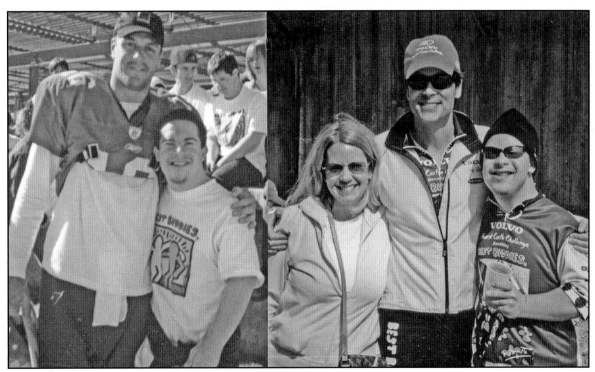

I have met two mayors and a governor, and many celebrities. From Jake Plummer to Rob Lowe.

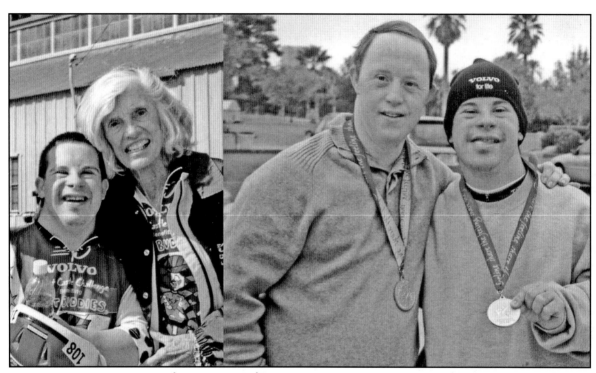

And my heroes, Eunice Kennedy Shriver
and Chris Burke. How cool is that?

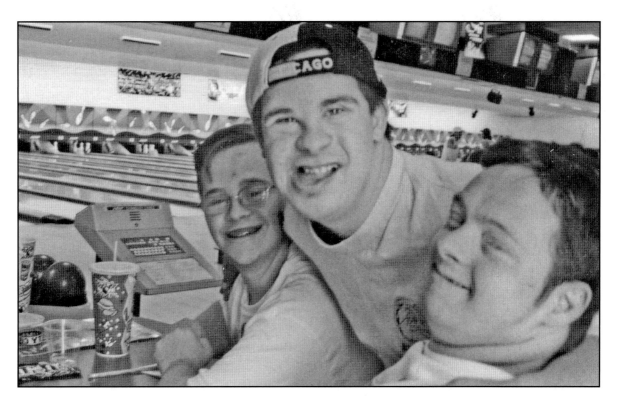

People called us Mongoloids. I think that's in China.

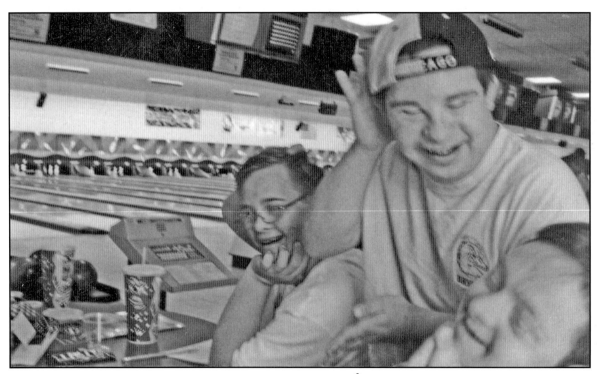

Yes our eyes are slanted.
Do all Chinese people have disabilities?

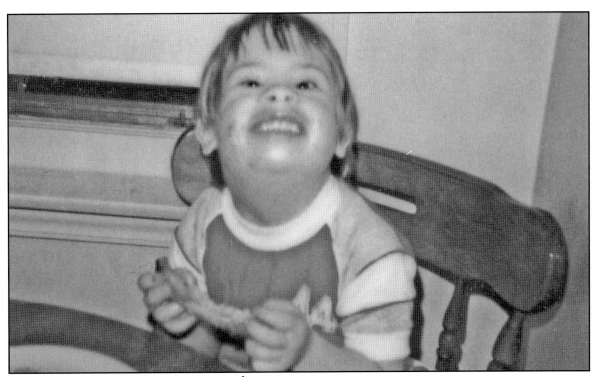

I am told I am retarded.
Gosh, I do not like that word.

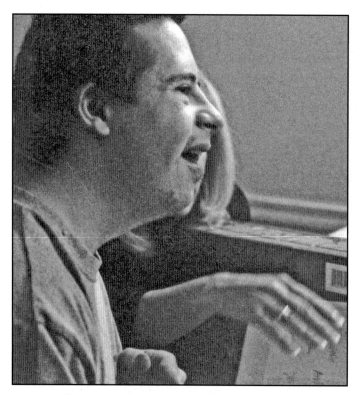

Can't you just come up to me
and say, "Hey, how is your day?"

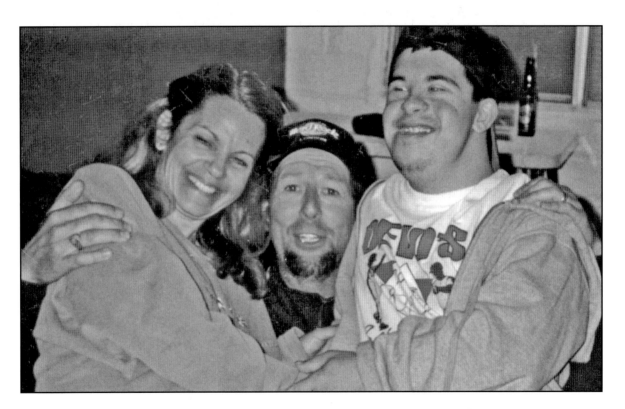

I have parents that I love. I love life.

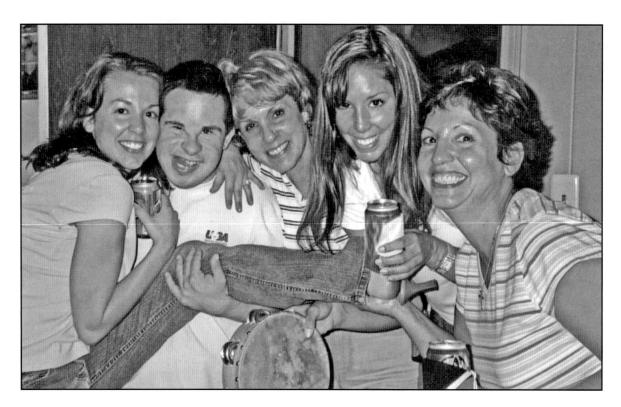

I have lots of relatives that I love. Isn't that normal?

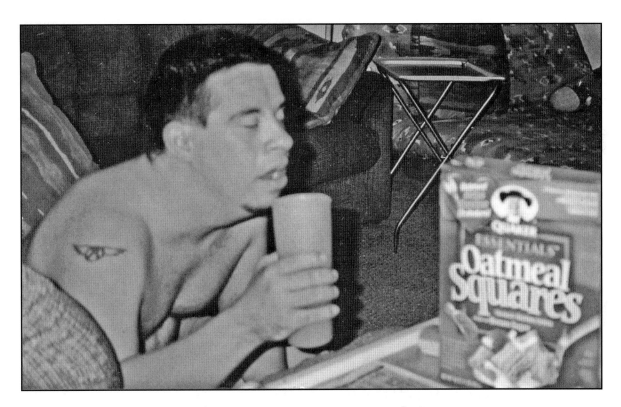

I wake up. I have breakfast.

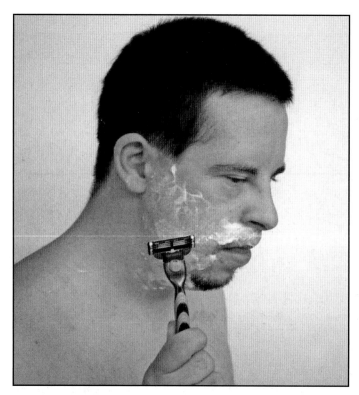

I shower and shave.
Sounds like normal.

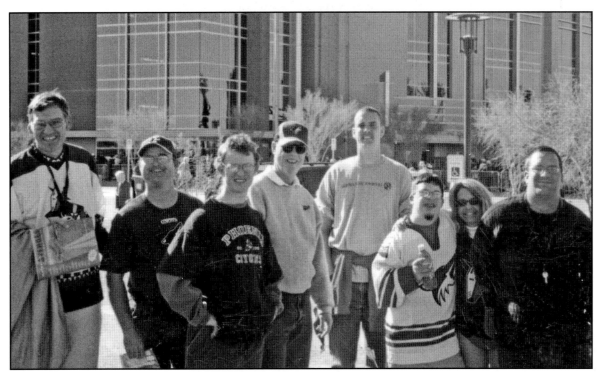

I have many friends.
We go to baseball and hockey games.

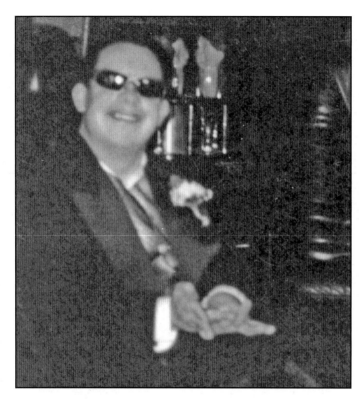

We go to movies and dances.
Still sounds normal.

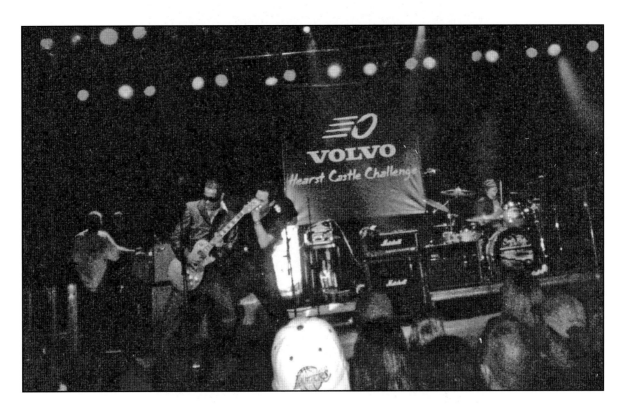

I go to concerts. I go shopping.

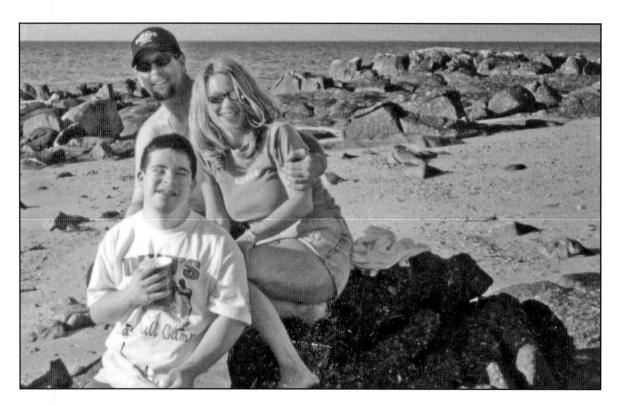

I go to the beach. Sound normal?

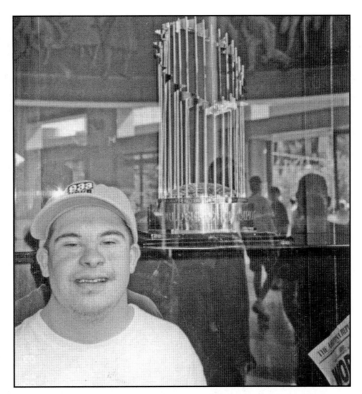

I dream. I hope. I have plans.
I have goals.

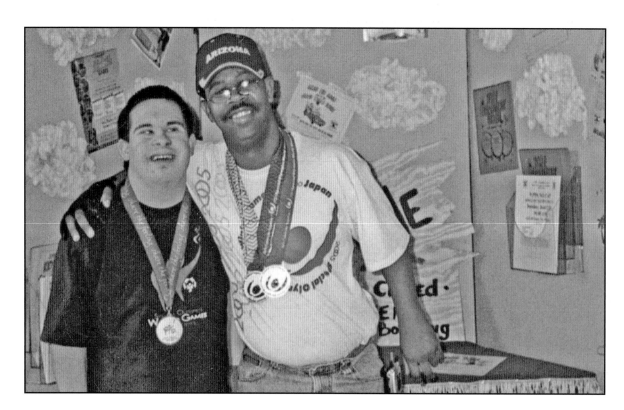

Isn't that normal? Or is it?

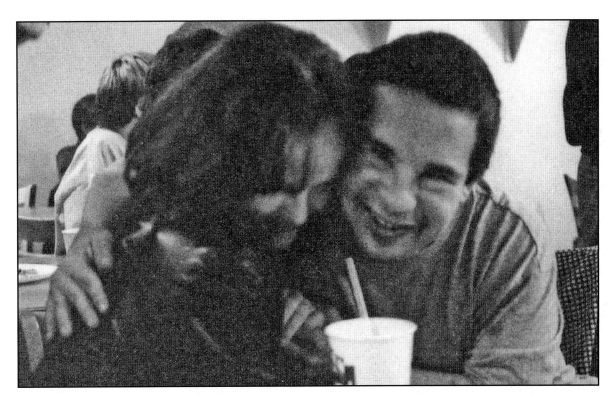

I don't lie. I don't cheat.

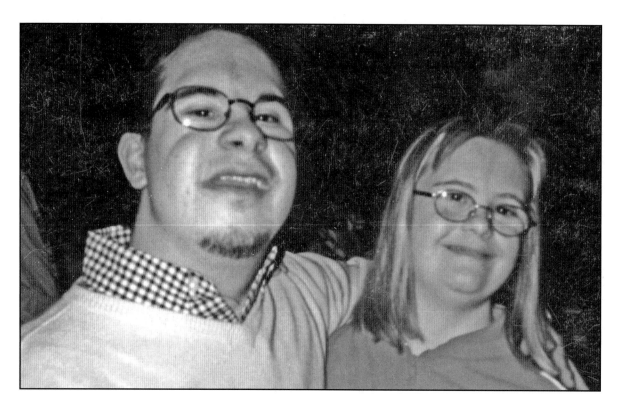

I don't steal. Now that's not normal.

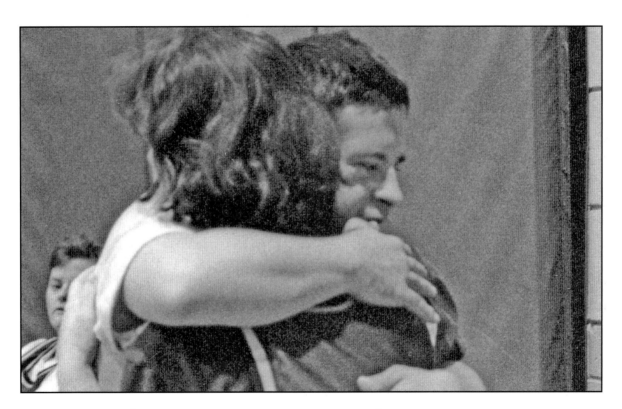

I don't try to deceive. I don't put on an act.

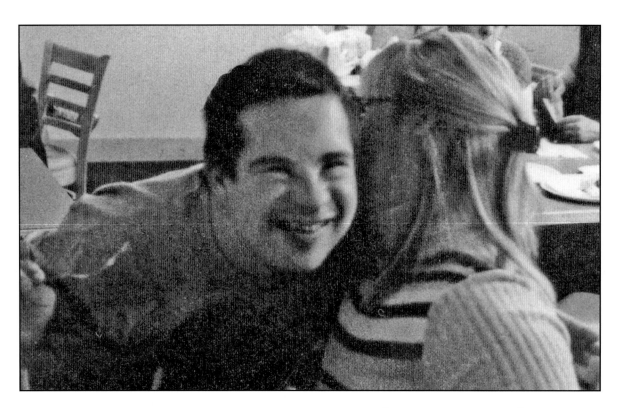

I just try to be me. Maybe I'm not normal.

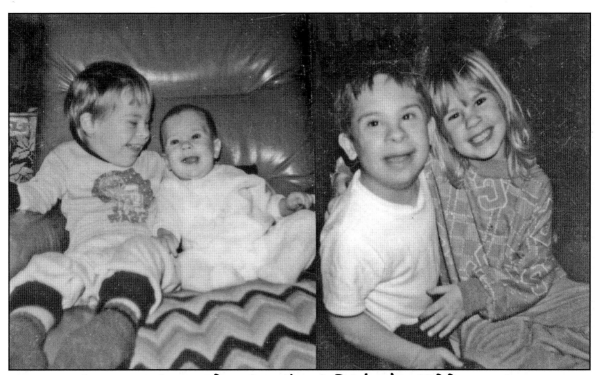

I am not perfect. Who is? I look different.
Doesn't everyone?

67

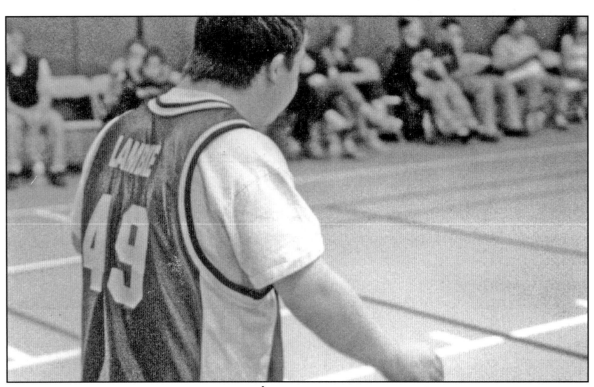

I just don't get it. Do you?
What is normal? I just am.

FIRST... SOME FACTS

Down Syndrome
Salvatore Tocci
2000 by Franklin Watts, Division of Grolier Publications Page 13

Dr. John Langdon Down, a British doctor, had been observing a large number of children who were mentally retarded. Some of these children had severe mental retardation, others were moderately retarded, and still others displayed only mild mental retardation. But what struck Dr. Down was what all these children had in common. He noticed the physical features that most of them shared. In a medical journal published in 1866, Dr. Down wrote, "Their hair is of a brownish colour, straight and scanty. The face is flat and broad. The cheeks are roundish. The eyes are obliquely placed. The forehead is wrinkled. The lips are large and thick. The tongue is long, thick, and is much roughened. The nose is small. The skin has a slightly yellowish tinge, and gives the appearance of being too large for the body. Dr. Down was the first to describe the features that are typical of people with a condition which is known today as Down syndrome. A syndrome is a collection of features or symptoms that characterize or indicate a disease or some abnormal condition. Because Dr. Down was the first to record the features in these children, the syndrome bears his name. Down syndrome is an abnormal condition marked by some degree of mental retardation and certain distinct physical features.

The hands of a child with Down syndrome are often smaller, and the fingers may be shorter. The fifth finger may curve inward slightly, having only one crease rather than the normal two. The palm of the hand often has only a single deep crease extending across the center. The feet are usually normal in both size and shape, but the space between the first and second toe may be quite large. The skin may be fair and have a spotted appearance. Children with Down syndrome usually have less hair than normal, and the hair may also be thin and soft. The child's eyes often appear to slant upward. Because of the Asian appearance caused by these slanted eyes, Down syndrome was once called "mongolism." In fact, Dr. Down referred to the "Mongolian type" in the paper he wrote in 1866. He attempted to find a connection between intelligence and race. He felt that because of their facial features, individuals with Down syndrome were part of a race of Asian people known as Mongols. Their mental retardation led Dr. Down to classify them as "idiots." Today, the term "mongoloid idiot" is obsolete and should never be used. Down syndrome has no relationship to any race, religion, or nationality. In addition, most people with Down syndrome have only mild to moderate mental retardation and thus cannot be classified as "idiots." Finally, people recognize that Down syndrome is NOT an indication that a person is severely mentally retarded, inferior, unhappy, or unable to function in society.

Not all children with Down syndrome will have all these physical traits. One child with Down syndrome might have only a few of these traits, while another child might have many. But three physical features are likely to be present in a child with Down syndrome: low muscle tone, upward-slanted eyes, and small ears. Another trait shared by almost all people with Down syndrome is a lower-than-normal intelligence.

MORE FACTS ABOUT DOWN SYNDROME

By Mary Bowman-Kruhm Ed. D.

GENETIC FORMS OF DOWN SYNDROME

A. Trisomy 21. There is an entire extra chromosome twenty-one in all cells. Most cases are this type – 95%.
B. Translocation is in about 4% of DS cases, the extra twenty-first chromosome material takes the place of part of another chromosome.
C. Mosaicism is in about 1% of people with DS, an extra whole chromosome is present, but only in some of the cells.

Some of the physical symptoms of DS may be milder in a child with mosaicism, since some of the child's cells are normal. Otherwise all three types are much the same in how they affect a baby born with DS.

IS DOWN SYNDROME INHERITED?

Most cases of DS are not inherited. Mothers or fathers do not cause it. No one can do anything to prevent it. Children with DS are born to people of all races, all countries, to both rich parents and poor. It is not caused by the health or diet of the parents or by anything that a mother does when she is pregnant. It is not a disease, and no one can catch it.

MEDICAL PROBLEMS ASSOCIATED WITH DOWN SYNDROME

- Between 40-60% of all infants with Down syndrome have some type of heart defect.
- Hypotonia (low muscle tone) is another common feature which is the cause of not only delayed gross motor development like crawling and walking, but also constipation and gastroesophageal reflux.
- Seizures occur in 5-10% of people with Down syndrome.
- Those with Down syndrome are at greater risk for leukemia, sleep apnea, hypothyroidism, celiac disease and diabetes.
- The prevalence of autism or autistic spectrum disorders is estimated to be between 5-7%.
- Atlantoaxial instability (AAI), which is caused by excess movement between the first and second vertebrae in the neck, occurs in approximately 15% of youths and causes a potential risk of spinal cord damage.

People with Down syndrome are active participants in the community; schools, jobs and leisure activities. Some live with family, some with friends and some independently.

At the beginning of the 20th century, there were close to 100,000 children in institutions— many of those were children with Down syndrome with a dismal existence and a life expectancy of 9 years. The gains made in the last third of the century in education, employment, and community living can, and must be, further broadened. The new century offers the possibility of unparalleled opportunities for individuals with Down syndrome. Life expectancy for a baby born today with Down syndrome is 55-60 years.

This is the first generation of individuals with Down syndrome to age. Many health care professionals are just beginning to understand what is "normal" aging and what may be certain conditions specific to Down syndrome. For example, there has been a tendency to over-diagnose Alzheimer's disease in those with Down syndrome because there is a close connection. Yet only 20-25% of all adults with Down syndrome show any of the dementia or cognitive decline that is the hallmark of Alzheimer's disease.

Research in Down syndrome is funded at an extremely low level compared to other disabilities. We must continue to increase funding since the key to also unlocking the problems associated with Down syndrome lies on the 21st chromosome. For example, current researchers say that raising the IQ points of an individual with Down syndrome by 20 points is not out of the question.

People with Down syndrome want to be accepted. They want to be included. They wish to be provided with choices and opportunities. People with Down syndrome have goals and dreams. They want to be heard and given the same respect as everyone else. Individuals with Down syndrome are thinking and feeling people, and they want to be treated as such. They want the same quality of life as everyone else.

Source: Mile High Down Syndrome Association (Colorado)

LANGUAGE GUIDELINES

"A person with Down syndrome is not a Downs."

The words that people use can help all individuals to lead more complete and enriching lives. Words can also create barriers and reinforce stereotypes. The primary goal of this statement is to ensure that correct language is used when talking, or writing about individuals with Down syndrome. The correct name of this diagnosis is Down syndrome. There is no apostrophe. The "s" in syndrome is not capitalized. An individual with Down syndrome is an individual first and foremost. The emphasis should be on the person, not the disability. Down syndrome is just one of many words that can be used to describe a person. A "child with Down syndrome" is a more appropriate way to discuss a person with this condition.

Words can create barriers. Try to recognize that a child is a "child with Down syndrome" or that an adult is "an adult with Down syndrome." A person with Down syndrome is not "a Downs." Children with Down syndrome grow into adults with Down syndrome; they do not remain "eternal children."

It is important to use the correct terminology. A person has mental retardation, rather than "suffers from," "is a victim of," "is diseased with," or "afflicted by."

Ask yourself if using the words "poor," "pitiful," or "unfortunate" when referring to an individual with Down syndrome is in his/her best interest. Each person has his/her own unique strength, capabilities, and talents. Try not to use the cliches that are so common when describing an individual with Down syndrome. To assume all people have the same characteristics or abilities is degrading. Also, it reinforces the stereotype that "All kids with Down syndrome are the same."

Most importantly, look at the person as an individual - your child, your family member, your student, and your friend. Proudly acknowledge his/her individuality and accomplishments.

(Language Guidelines compiled by the Down Syndrome Society of Rhode Island and reprinted with their permission.)

DID YOU KNOW...

- There are more than 350,000 individuals in the United States with Down syndrome
- Down syndrome occurs in approximately one in every 800 to 1,000 births
- Around 80% of babies with Down syndrome are born to mothers under the age of 35
- National Down Syndrome Society is one of the largest non-government supporters of Down syndrome research in the world
- National Down Syndrome Society established October as National Down Syndrome Awareness Month
- National Down Syndrome Society has been helping people with Down syndrome and their families for 25 years

WELCOME TO HOLLAND

by Emily Perl Kingsley

I am often asked to describe the experience of raising a child with a disability – to try to help people who have not shared that unique experience to understand it, to imagine how it would feel. It's like this...

When you're going to have a baby, it's like planning a fabulous vacation trip – to Italy. You buy a bunch of guide books and make your wonderful plans. The Coliseum. The Michelangelo David. The gondolas in Venice. You may learn some handy phrases in Italian. It's all very exciting.

After months of eager anticipation, the day finally arrives. You pack your bags and off you go. Several hours later, the plane lands. The stewardess comes in and says, "Welcome to Holland."

"Holland?!?" you say. "What do you mean Holland?? I signed up for Italy! I'm supposed to be in Italy. All my life I've dreamed of going to Italy."

But there's been a change in the flight plan. They've landed in Holland and there you must stay.

The important thing is that they haven't taken you to a horrible, disgusting, filthy place, full of pestilence, famine and disease. It's just a different place.

So you must go out and buy new guide books. And you must learn a whole new language. And you will meet a whole new group of people you would never have met.

It's just a different place. It's slower-paced than Italy, less flashy than Italy. But after you've been there for a while and you catch your breath, you look around... and you begin to notice that Holland has windmills... and Holland has tulips. Holland even has Rembrandts.

But everyone you know is busy coming and going from Italy... and they're all bragging about what a wonderful time they had there. And for the rest of your life, you will say "Yes, that's where I was supposed to go. That's what I had planned."

And the pain of that will never, ever, ever, ever go away... because the loss of that dream is a very very significant loss.

But... if you spend your life mourning the fact that you didn't get to Italy, you may never be free to enjoy the very special, the very lovely things... about Holland.

ENDORSEMENTS

Tom Lambke's latest book, "I Just Am," perfectly illustrates the essence of what it means to have Down syndrome, and I couldn't be more pleased that he is getting the word out. Tom's passion, dedication, and commitment to assisting people with disabilities is unmatched. He is hardworking and very creative. He is making a difference, because, he "just is" too.

Janet Giel-Romo
President of DSNetwork Arizona
Reading Specialist at Carl Hayden High School
Special Education Teacher at Carl Hayden High School

When I was asked to write something for Bryan's book I struggled. Knowing Bryan and having worked with him in my professional capacity led my thoughts in a direction that did not satisfactorily explain the experience of Bryan. On my third read of this book, I realized what was missing. I was trying to talk about Bryan from a professional perspective. While that reference point is accurate, it is inadequate and insufficient to portray Mr. Bryan Lambke. So, let me try again. I had the pleasure to work with and to come to know Bryan, during his high school years. Bryan has a dynamic spirit and takes on the challenges that life presents to us all, as well as those that are uniquely his, with courage, humor and determination. Bryan infects those around him with his joy and exuberance. Bryan demonstrates the theme of this book every moment of his life. Bryan is a capable human being who is as normal and as abnormal as the rest of us. He is just like you and me: he sees his world in a unique and different way and at the same time, just as we do. The range of human variation is wide enough that it encompasses Einstein and Mozart and Lance Armstrong and average mere mortals like Bryan and like you and me. I applaud Bryan and his family in bringing our sameness and difference to the page. It seems less important after all, how tall, or rich or smart someone is, than whether he or she is a person of courage, compassion, humor and heart.

Steven N. Shively, Ph.D.
School Psychologist at Corona del Sol High School
2005 Arizona School Psychologist of the Year

This book provides a wonderful glimpse into Bryan's life and provides insight about the uniqueness and sameness of us all. To honor diversity, we must celebrate our similarities. Bryan and his family share a brief view into "uniqueness," while sharing the human qualities, emotions, and dreams we all share. I would share this book with families of children with Down syndrome as it reinforces determination, love and support. It includes valuable information in an easy to read and understandable format.

Dr. Patty Vogel
Director of Educational Services
Tempe Union High School District

I laughed and cried through "I Just Am." Your book, told honestly and without ego, is about the lifelong struggle to convey to others who you are and how you see the world. It is a book that can change ignorance and typecasting. As I read parts to my daughter, she exclaimed, "Oh! I never knew Bryan felt just like me!" Thank you for writing your story, Bryan.

TaMarla Forrest
Special Education Department Chair
formerly Bryan's Special Education Teacher
Corona del Sol High School, Tempe, AZ

The greatest gift our children teach us is to have unconditional love. Bryan Lambke has taught his father well what it means to truly love and accept all people for who they are.

Gina Johnson
President/Founder
Sharing Down Syndrome Arizona Inc.

My name is Jamaica Ballard and I am a Special Education Teacher in the Tempe Union High School District. I read the book, "I Just Am" and felt a strong sense of love and understanding. My brother has severe and multiple disabilities and I know firsthand what the Lambke's have experienced. The story inspired me and gave me a great sense of pride. It was gratifying to hear Bryan's personal journeys from his perspective. Bryan is a bright light who shines every time I see him smile. The best part of the book was seeing Bryan's pictures accompany his words. I would like to thank Bryan and his family for sharing their story. This book is a celebration of family, life and love.

with warmest regards,
Jamaica Ballard
Tempe/Kyrene CEC Special Educator of the Year 2002-2003
Special Olympics World Games Track and Field Coach 2003 Governing Board Award for Excellence Tempe Union High School District 2004-2005

I JUST AM is an extraordinary, honest and real-life look at a young man's journey as he over-comes great obstacles to achieve incredible feats.

Mark Villa
Former Chandler Therapeutic Recreation Program Coordinator
and Chandler Special Olympics Head Coach
Future Special Education Teacher - Elementary School

Book Order Form

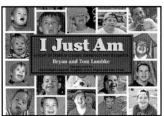

I Just Am

A STORY OF DOWN SYNDROME AWARENESS AND TOLERANCE

Bryan and Tom Lambke

with a foreword by
Shannon D. R. Ringenbach, Ph.D.
Department of Kinesiology Arizona
State University
and introduction by
Cheryl Rogers-Barnett, daughter of
Roy Rogers and Dale Evans

Name: _____

Address: _____

City: _____

State: _____ Zip: _____

Daytime Phone: _____ Fax: _____

E-Mail: _____

Method of payment

❑ Check ❑ Visa ❑ MasterCard

❑ Discover Card ❑ American Express

Account Number: _____

Expiration Date: _____

Signature: _____

One book is $14.99.

Order 2 or more and get free shipping.*

Order 4 or more and receive 10% off plus free shipping.*

Shipping and Handling: 15% of the total order.

*Ground shipping only. Allow 1 to 2 weeks for delivery.

❑ *Yes, please send me a Five Star Publications catalog.*

How were you referred to Five Star Publications?

❑ Friend ❑ Internet ❑ Book Show ❑ Other

Item	Quantity	Unit price	Total Price
Subtotal			
Shipping			
I bought 2 or more—ship it to me FREE!			
TOTAL			

Mail or Fax your order to: Five Star Publications, Inc.,
P.O. Box 6698, Chandler, AZ 85246-6698
Fax: 480-940-8787 Phone: 480-940-8182 Toll free: 866-471-0777

www.FiveStarPublications.com • www.IJustAm.org

86